Keto Diet

*A Beginner's Guide to Better Health
and Weight Loss*

By Michael Lane

content within this book has been derived from various sources. Please consult a licensed professional before attempting any techniques outlined in this book.

By reading this document, the reader agrees that under no circumstances are is the author responsible for any losses, direct or indirect, which are incurred as a result of the use of information contained within this document, including, but not limited to, —errors, omissions, or inaccuracies.

Table of Contents

Introduction...7

Chapter One: What is the Ketogenic Diet?.........11

Ketosis..16

Chapter Two: Is the Keto Diet Right for You?....19

Precautions...21

Chapter Three: Keto Diet vs. Atkins vs. Paleo....23

Paleo Diet...23

Keto Diet..25

Atkins Diet...25

Chapter Four: Keto Diet Benefits and Side Effects...33

Side Effects..37

Hypoglycemia...38

HPA Axis Dysfunction....................................39

Keto breath...42

*Chapter Five: Foods to Eat and Foods to Avoid.*44

Foods to Avoid...44

Foods to eat..46

How To Get Started?..52

Overview of the Keto Diet..................................56

Chapter Six: 5 Examples of Meals/Recipes Allowed on the Ketogenic Diet.........................64

Breakfast..65

Keto Blueberry Pancakes................................66

Keto Coconut Pancakes..................................67

Lunch...68

Keto frittata...69

Dinner..70

Keto Meatloaf 70

Keto dessert 71

Keto Brownies 72

Chapter Seven: Tracking Macros and Counting Calories *74*

Intermittent Fasting and the Keto Diet 76

Exercise while on the Keto diet 83

Chapter Eight: Exercising on the Keto Diet *88*

For Overweight People Trying to Lose Weight 88

For Those Who Lift Weights 89

For Those Who Practice High-Intensity Sports Or Activities 90

Chapter Nine: Following the Keto Diet While Traveling or Eating Out *94*

Conclusion *100*

References *102*

Introduction

I want to thank you for choosing this book, 'Keto Diet: A Beginner's Guide to Better Health and Weight loss' and hope you find the book informative and interesting.

Health should be the first and foremost thing at the top of your list of priorities. There is always time to work hard and be successful, but if you don't pay your body its due attention, you cannot possibly enjoy all that you work hard for. Out of all the ailments that are caused due to the negligence of health, one of the most common is obesity or being overweight.

Over the years, there have been too many food choices for people to pick and eat. We don't check what we eat or how often and just let our body take it all in; however, there is a limit for your body to tolerate such things. Too much food will inadvertently lead to excessive weight gain. And most of these foods contain substances that are not healthy. At some point, you realize how your clothes don't fit or how lazy you feel all the time and need to take a thorough look at the state you have put your body in. This is when the regret kicks in and you try all the fad diets out there that claim to help you lose weight in a week.

This is not the approach you should take. Especially when it comes to health and losing weight, it is not about quick fixes. You could try starving for a week or only drinking liquids, and you might see the number on the scale go down a little, but what about later when you go back to your old food habits? Do you think the numbers will stay the same? Fad diets don't work most of the time and more often than not, they will harm your health rather than benefit you. Instead, why not try something that actually works?

In this book, you will read everything you need to know about the ketogenic diet. You might already have heard of it or this might be the first time you came across the keto diet concept. Here you will learn how you can include the ketogenic diet as a part of your lifestyle and how it will benefit you. It is not about starving yourself but giving your body the right kind of food in the right quantities. Unlike other fad diets, the keto diet will show you real results that will last over time. The book discusses in detail about getting started on the diet and following it in the right manner so you get optimal results.

The keto diet advocates the concept of eating like our ancestors used to. They did not overeat and get fat and sit around counting calories to lose weight. The food industry has been the main culprit behind our deteriorating health and eating habits over the years. All the different products they provide might seem to be convenient and tempting but it is at the cost of our good health. We are hardly conscious of the ingredients of all the things we consume and do not consider how it affects our body. It is high time that we do so. Instead of consuming unhealthy processed food that is laden with chemicals and very little nutrition, we should go back to the basics. Eating as our ancestors did might just be the solution to most of our issues.

Stop listening to those who advocate unhealthy fad diets and just start eating better. You don't have to cut out all fat from your diet. For some reason, most people have tried to blame all health issues on fat, but fat is actually a crucial part of your diet and your body needs it, albeit in the appropriate amount. One of the main culprits that you should really focus on eliminating from your diet is sugar. This one ingredient is the cause of most health issues and obesity in people.

In the keto diet, you will learn what your body really needs and how you don't have to stop eating all the food you enjoy. I have also provided a few ketogenic recipes that will help you get started with the diet. You can also add your own ketogenic twist to your regular recipes, as long as you use keto-compliant ingredients. To make it easy for you, I have listed the foods that you should eat and avoid while on the diet.

As you read on, keep an open mind and try it out for yourself. Once you see results yourself, you will understand why the keto diet is actually effective.

Thank you once again for choosing this book. I hope it helps you embark on your weight loss journey.

Chapter One:
What is the Ketogenic Diet?

The keto or ketogenic diet is unlike fad diets and is more of a type of lifestyle. The diet does not set rules for not eating or just eating a cup of vegetables or drinking juice in order to lose weight. It is not a taxing diet that will ask you to exert immense control and cut off all the food you like in exchange for fruits and vegetables. The keto diet does not ask you to starve yourself for days at a time either. Instead, the diet will help you understand how your food habits have turned bad over the years and what you can do to regain your health. You will learn that all your excess weight is there not just because of overeating and not exercising.

Research and basic science actually prove that it is not true. All excessive weight and health problems are due to eating the wrong kinds of food, and not just how much. The food industry provides us with innumerable options of food, most of which are not nutritious but instead detrimental to our health. There is a reason why most grandparents seem to be unsatisfied with the diets that this generation follows. Even up to a few decades ago, it was not as bad as it is these days. Our ancestors ate much healthier and wholesome foods and not processed unhealthy meals. There are no substitutes for the real food that our body needs. Most of the food choices we make these days are based on incorrect facts and so those that are told to us in order to lose weight. You don't need to count calories for every meal or hit the gym twice a day. Instead, you need to learn what is right and wrong for your body and start eating accordingly.

It is important to remember that everything you hear is not true. A lot of negativity has been attached to fats over the years even though it is not the main culprit behind obesity and related conditions. The naturally occurring fats that are found in meat, dairy or fish are actually healthy and have been a part of the human diet since the beginning of our existence. It is only in the past couple of decades that fat has been labeled as bad and prohibited if you want to stay fit.

The real culprit is actually the food industry and all the processed food that it has pushed for profit at the cost of good health. Around the 1970's everyone started being told that fat was unhealthy and more low-fat food products were sold; however, you will see that the average weight of people also started increasing around that same time. The number of type two diabetes cases also saw a spike and this disease is nearly always related to excessive weight. Before this era, diabetes was actually quite uncommon. Should you really be blaming all fatty food for the problems created by processed food? Although we now have more options for low fat, low calorie, etc. types of food, our generation has a lower life expectancy than any of our ancestors. This is despite all the advancements in medicine and is solely caused by our unhealthy diet.

Sugar is one of the main ingredients in the modern diet that harms us. A little amount of sugar does not harm anyone but there is no real nutritional value to it. If you consume too much of sugar, you will see rapid weight gain, medical conditions and general lethargy in everything you do. Refined sugars constitute a large part of most modern food items like packaged juices, sodas, etc. and it has to be stopped. Excess sugar in our body is converted to fat and leads to more weight gain. When people started looking for easier alternatives for preparing meals, the food industry produced thousands of new products for consumption. They gained enough power to influence how people look at food. The food pyramid that is taught to us since school is also influenced by it where they place fats as the worst choice. It was just used as a way for the food corporations to profit more from consumers.

Once people took notice of how fast they are gaining weight, they started trying fad diets that claim to help them lose weight very quickly. You can choose to starve yourself for a week, or just eat boiled vegetables, or go through a liquid diet and many other such fad diets. None of these, however, are healthy or sustainable in the long term.

The best option that we recommend is to go back to how our ancestors ate. This is where the keto diet helps you. In this book, you will learn to understand how your food is really processed by your body and what you should eat accordingly. Instead of listening to others, think for yourself and do what is good for your body. The food industry has demonized fats but our body actually needs carbohydrates far less comparatively.

If you want to eat as people did in the old days, one of the main ingredients you need to reduce or cut out is sugar. Back then, they did not have access to any refined carbohydrates and were healthier due to this. Basic grains like wheat are also grown very differently in modern breeding methods and this changes their constituents. The original form of all foods is the most nutritious. Fad diets usually ask you to cut out fat but it is crucial for many functions in the human body.

When you try out fad diets, you are so busy calorie counting that most of the time you don't eat enough and are left hungry. This will inadvertently lead you to give up and binge out on food. Fat helps by satiating your appetite. It takes longer to digest and thus keeps your hunger at bay for longer than with carbs. Carbohydrates get broken down quickly and leave you hungry again right after a meal.

The high sugar content in most carb foods cause spikes in adrenalin levels and lead to diabetes very often. The ketogenic diet guides you to eat healthy fats from meat, dairy, nuts, etc. and a moderate amount of protein that is healthy for you. The carbohydrate content in a keto diet is extremely reduced. You need to increase your fat consumption in a keto diet in order to keep your body in the ketosis state and lose weight.

The ketogenic diet advocates very low

amounts of carbohydrates. It demonstrates how you can eat and push your body into a fat burning cycle while still consuming fat. You can look into it and see how thousands of people have tried the keto diet and benefited from it in terms of health, stamina, weight loss, etc.

The "keto" here is derived from ketones in our body that are the fuel molecules in our body. When the glucose or blood sugar level in your body is low, your body will use ketones as the alternative source of energy it requires. When you consume very little amounts of carbohydrates, they quickly get broken into blood sugar and along with the proteins in your diet, your body will produce ketones. You need to remember that the protein levels also need to be in moderate amounts. The fat in the liver is used to produce these ketones, which then act as a fuel source for the entire body. Ketones are especially useful as a source of energy for the brain that is constantly functioning.

The only alternative that the brain has for fuel other than glucose is ketones. When you follow a ketogenic diet, instead of glucose, your body switches to fat as its fuel source. It gets accustomed to your diet and starts burning fat all the time in order to provide sufficient energy to your body. The insulin levels in your body dip low and the fat burning process becomes even faster. This is how the keto diet makes it easy for the body to start accessing stored fats and burning them off. You will soon see yourself losing any excess weight and also start noticing how your health improves in other aspects. The state where your body produces many ketones is called ketosis. Ketosis is a metabolic process that is initiated quickly especially when you are fasting. This is why intermittent fasting can also benefit you on this diet and it is explained further in the book.

Ketosis

Ketosis is the keyword in the ketogenic diet. It is a metabolic process where your body uses stored fat instead of glucose for energy. Burning off stored fat is how you can easily lose weight by following a ketogenic diet. Ketosis is a natural state in the body that you induce further by consuming more fats than carbohydrates in this diet. Your body will always try to adapt to how you feed and treat it. When you consume more fats, it will automatically start using fats for energy in the ketosis state. Your liver will produce more ketones and fat will be the main energy source now instead of glucose. As the body requires more energy, it will start utilizing the fat stored all around the body. At this point, you will see a difference in the appearance of your body.

The part of your brain that controls hunger is naturally conditioned to be sated by fat, so when you consume more of it, you stay full for longer and don't suffer from hunger pangs. This part is where most diets fail and leave you hungry. There is only a certain amount of willpower that you can have to control such hunger so you will probably end up overeating later to make up for that hungry state. Such binge eating always involves carb-loaded foods that are converted to fat and stored in your body.

Unlike these diets, the keto diet will help you feel full and still keep burning fat all day. As you get used to the diet, you will slowly learn to sustain it for a longer time. One question that comes up while considering the ketogenic diet is about cholesterol. You might wonder if all the fat will cause your cholesterol levels to rise and block your arteries. This is not true. Ketosis causes an increase in the good kind of cholesterol that is HDL. The cholesterol that should be lessened in your body is LDL. Hence, when your body is in ketosis, the HDL levels rise and this cholesterol actually functions to take LDL to the liver for processing.

Cholesterol is not all bad; certain levels are essential in the body. You need to consider which foods will cause an increase in the bad type of LDL cholesterol. Instead of cholesterol, your focus should be on avoiding too much carbohydrates that are the main culprit for most unhealthy conditions. Over the years, studies have been done to see how ketosis and the keto diet affect people in different areas of life. In sportsmen, the keto diet has actually shown to help increase their endurance.

Previously, they used carb loading to provide their body with energy to endure long periods of sports; however, you now understand that carbs burn faster and they can only provide energy for a certain period of time. Fats, on the other hand, take longer to burn and provide energy for longer periods. This has shown to be more beneficial for such athletes. Ketosis also helps improve focus and mental stamina.

A lot of research is still being done to validate the scientific value of the keto diet and prove its benefit for people; however, it has shown to help many people in losing weight and is a much healthier alternative to other diets. A keto diet can be continued for a long time as a lifestyle change that will benefit you.

Chapter Two:
Is the Keto Diet Right for You?

Although I recommend the ketogenic diet, the results may vary from person to person. While following this or any other diet, you need to know what is suitable for you. You will need to ask yourself some questions before you decide to get started.

Firstly, this diet is more beneficial for people who are solely looking to lose excess fat from their body at first. Whether you want to lose a small or large amount of body fat, the keto diet can work well for this purpose. Hence it is more appropriate for overweight or obese people.

If you are on another diet or have previously tried other diets, consider how you feel while on it. Do you keep feeling hungry and crave more food? This is quite probable if you eat carb-loaded meals. You might eat a huge dinner but within an hour or so you will crave a snack while on such diets. The keto diet will benefit you in this case because it helps to control hunger pangs and will regulate your blood sugar and insulin levels.

Due to a habitual diet, some people don't feel satisfied with their meals unless they include heavy carbs. They always need some bread or rice or other carbs on their plate. People such as these compulsively eat carbs in order to achieve that bloated feeling that carbs provide; however, it is a very unhealthy way to eat. Loading up on fats instead of carbs will give you the same satisfaction or better but in a healthier way. You will also stay full for longer because fats take longer to burn off than carbs.

The keto diet works for both lazy and disciplined people. It is up to you to decide if you want a strict or more easygoing keto diet. Some people like to work on instinct when considering the food they eat while others prefer specific markers set for what their meals should consist of. This adjustable aspect of the keto diet makes it suitable for all types of people.

A ketogenic diet will slowly help you get rid of bad food habits. The processed food diet most people follow cause untimely cravings. There are people who feel quite restless if they don't have certain snacks or sweets every single day. This unhealthy food addiction can be very damning for the body and mostly consists of empty calories. Once you start reducing the carbohydrates in your diet and eating more fats, you will slowly get your body accustomed to breaking off the carb addiction. This will help you lose fat and maintain a healthy weight long-term.

It is easy to stick to a keto diet because the main parts of the meal such as meat, fish, and vegetables are not prohibited. The diet is only difficult for those who are too dependent on bread or such starchy foods in their meals. People who are overweight usually have a problem staying motivated to continue a diet. This is why strict diets often result in failure, but the keto diet can be a bit simpler for you compared to these diets. Keep track of your results in the first couple of weeks where you will first lose water weight. Slowly you will see the fat shedding from all parts of your body. Progress will be the best motivation for you to stay on the diet long-term.

The ketogenic diet is especially recommended for those suffering from type 2 diabetes. This disease can cause a lot of health issues but is reversible if you follow the right diet. The keto diet helps to eliminate all sugar and carbs from your diet so your blood glucose levels are regulated. Within the first few months of following the keto diet itself, you will see improvement in your condition. It is very important to stay away from sugar in this condition and the keto diet already tells you how it affects you negatively.

The keto diet will work for you only if you stay dedicated for long enough. Unlike other fad diets, it does not promise you instant gratifying results. The goal is more long-term and so you need to stay patient and watch as it works on your body. If you really want to see improvement in your health you should try the keto diet and stick to it till you see results.

Precautions

Just like any other diet, consult a doctor before you follow the ketogenic diet. Your body is different from others and has its own special needs. There are certain conditions in which a particular diet might not be suitable for you. This is why a health screen is necessary to determine if you should follow the ketogenic diet or not.

The ketogenic diet is not recommended for people with kidney, liver or pancreatic diseases. There are other conditions like muscular dystrophy as well, which make it unsuitable for those people. If you have type 1 diabetes, the keto diet is completely unsuitable for you. In the case of diabetes type 2, it works for some and is not appropriate for others. You should consult your doctor to determine this. If you have gestational diabetes as well, keto is not the diet for you.

Women who are pregnant or nursing are also recommended to stay away from such diets. Such conditions require very healthy and nutritious diets and need to be accommodating to the child as well. People who suffer from eating disorders also need to be more careful about any diet they try. It is more important to focus on teaching healthy eating habits first. Going on any strict diet might not be helpful.

As you can see, there are certain conditions that make a particular diet unsuitable for your body. The goal is to help your body stay healthy and reach an appropriate weight using the right diet for you. As long as you don't suffer from the above-mentioned conditions, the keto diet will definitely be a good choice for you.

Chapter Three:
Keto Diet vs. Atkins vs. Paleo

When you are on the lookout for the right diet for you, you can actually get quite confused. There are so many different diets out there these days, which all claim to give you quick and effective results. Each one of the diets claim to guarantee weight loss and improve your body; however, if you really look into them, you will see most are just fads, some are not effective at all and some not enough. One of the common factors amongst these ineffective diets is how restrictive they are and how they demotivate the person from following through with them.

There are a few diets that are based on more scientific research and have proven to be quite effective for different people around the world. Amongst all the diets that have gained popularity these days and are said to really work, the keto diet, Paleo diet, and the Atkins diet are particularly prominent. Let's take a look at the features of each of these diets and how they differ from each other. You will see that they are all actually quite similar with overlapping features.

Paleo Diet

The Paleo diet is also known as the caveman diet and is derived from the term "Paleolithic". This diet advises you to eat only food that was available to our ancestors in the Paleolithic era. It gives you a general idea of what you should eat if you consider only foods that were available in the early ages. This rules out any processed foods, fast food, ready-to-eat meals, packaged food, etc. You need to imagine what a caveman would have available to him like raw meat or vegetables or fruits and stick to these while preparing your meals.

Scientists who approve of the Paleo diet argue that cavemen or our ancestors were much healthier than we are and did not suffer from many modern diseases like obesity that are prominent now. They attribute this good health to their healthy diet. The Paleo diet, therefore, has no room for chips and burgers and butter and sodas. Life was very simple back in the Paleolithic era, at least if you consider the food aspect. They just ate from whatever they could find in their surroundings. There were no supermarkets, canned food, or any processed food at all. It is easy to imagine that era and avoid any such food on the Paleo diet. It is definitely healthier if you just eat and cook fresh meat and vegetables. There are no hidden preservatives or additives in these compared to processed food.

There are also those who criticize the Paleo diet because they believe that the human digestive system has changed in the past thousands of years and adapted to the modern diet. The supporters believe otherwise and think that we are still suited for the Paleolithic diet. If you want to try the Paleo diet, stock up on eggs, fish, meat, fruits, vegetables, nuts, seeds any naturally occurring ingredients. Get rid of any refined sugar, cakes, and pastries, legumes, dairy, grains, vegetable oils, alcohol, processed food, etc. Try growing your own produce if you really can.

Keto Diet

You probably have a better idea of the keto diet from the rest of this book and it doesn't really need an introduction anymore. Out of the three diets, the keto diet is the most technical but has the largest following due to its effective results. The unconventional approach of this diet makes some people doubt it but this is what made it effective. This diet also advocates eating more wholesome food as our ancestors did but not necessarily as far back as the Paleolithic era.

The keto diet depends on the process of ketosis to lose excess stored fat. It also requires a reduction in carbohydrate consumption while fats are increased. Originally, the diet was tried in order to study the effect on epileptic children and there were positive results.

Atkins Diet

The Atkins diet is a bit more complex than

the Paleo or Keto diet. The technical nature of this diet makes it a little harder to convince people to try it. This means that not everyone can understand or follow it; however, for someone who is considering the ketogenic diet, this can be used as a trial before they follow the strict keto rules. The concept of the Atkins food chart is ketogenic but not as strict as the keto diet. It is named after the cardiologist Robert Coleman Atkins who conceptualized it; however, it also places a restriction on the consumption of carbohydrates but does not give specifics in terms of quantity of the carbohydrates.

Although it talks of how carbohydrates need to be reduced from the diet, it is not as focused on restrictions as the ketogenic diet and hence not as quick with results. The Atkins diet also suggests that you can reduce carbs when you are trying to lose weight but increase them back a little when you achieve a set goal. In the keto diet, you are asked to keep the carb content in your diet low at all times.

The disadvantage of the Atkins diet toward the end is that you increase the carb intake a lot but your body is not accustomed to ketosis. Because of this excess carb intake, you might experience lethargy and feel unwell most of the time. The Atkins diet was actually extremely popular when it was first introduced but then the hype died down; however, it is still famous enough that better versions of it are still brought forward from time to time to let people try it.

While comparing the three diets, there are

certain factors you will notice that will help you decide which is more appropriate for you to follow.

Firstly, you need to consider which is the easiest and most difficult for you to follow. You have to read labels carefully while you are on the keto and Atkins diet in particular. Carefully assess any ingredients you add to your meals especially when you buy packaged products. In terms of consistency, you need to make sure that you don't increase your carb intake above 35g in the keto diet per day. In Atkins, you can be more flexible and have more carbs if you want.

It can depend on how much weight you want to lose and how fast. Such details are of little importance in these two diets. In the Paleo diet, you don't have to think much, just eat simple foods that you could imagine cavemen eating and avoid the rest. Natural foods make it a lot easier to help you lose weight.

If you want to compare the diets according to how effective they are, you have to remember that each has its own benefits and results differ from person to person. One diet might be highly effective for one person but not so much for another person. Also, most healthy diets won't give you quick results that will motivate you to stick to the diet. Patience and persistence are crucial for long-term results. At the very least, try a diet for a month or two to see how it works for you. If you see absolutely no change, you can consider switching over to another, but this should only be if you are properly following the diet in the first place. In general, all three of these diets are usually effective for people.

There are some who try to avoid the ketogenic diet due to skepticism about consuming more fat but research has shown that it is an effective diet. For those who need more carbs in their diet like athletes, Atkins is more appropriate compared to the keto diet. The Paleo diet will help you lose weight but maybe not as quickly as Atkins or Keto diet. You can decide on your diet depending on how soon you expect results and what you prefer eating.

In terms of popularity, many want to go for the tried and tested method. People want to try a diet that many others say have tried and found to be effective. Many people also follow diets just because their favorite celebrity endorsed it. Popular diets are a little easier to follow because you can even join support groups related to them. Like I said before, remember that different diets work for different people. Don't compare your progress with someone else's.

Your end goal is another thing that will help you differentiate and choose a diet. For those who cannot count calories or pay attention to details in the long run, the Paleo diet is the easiest option. It is very flexible as long as you just eat wholesome natural foods. It gives you a healthy diet and helps you to lose weight with long-term benefits and very few side effects if any. The ketogenic and Atkins diet might not be something you can follow for a long time unless you are very disciplined but are the preferred choice if you want to really lose excess weight. Overall, let's see how these three diets differ from each other:

•	The keto diet and Atkins diet are effective for weight loss and the Paleo diet is recommended for better health.

•	The keto diet is very strict in terms of fats and carbs ratio while the Atkins diet is less so. The Paleo diet has no such restrictions at all.

•	All three of the diets tend to give you some flu-like side effects in the initial adaptation stage.

•	The Paleo diet is more popular than the keto diet, which is more common than the Atkins diet.

•	The main benefit of the keto diet is fat loss; the Atkins diet is easier than the keto diet in achieving ketosis and the Paleo diet has the most different types of food choices.

•	The main downside of the keto diet is the strict restrictions on carbohydrates. The problem with the Atkins diet is that it is not always effective compared to the other two. The Paleo diet is ineffective in terms of focused weight loss.

The one common thing amongst all three diets is that they all advocate a restriction on the consumption of processed foods and sugar. This is because there is scientific proof that most processed products have hidden ingredients that are harmful to our body and not nutritional at all. Sugar is a particularly harmful ingredient in the modern diet that has no nutritional value, causes weight gain and leads to other medical conditions. Hence, no matter which of these diets you try, they will all ask you to eat more wholesome food.

You also need to remember that any diet is difficult to begin with unless you can endure a little during the transition phase. Your mind and body take time to come to terms with any changes. The initial side effects are just your body's way of reacting to these changes but these are temporary and can be easily dealt with. After the initial adaptation phase, you will start feeling healthier and notice changes in a matter of time. If you keep risk factors in mind, Paleo is definitely the safest and healthiest bet for a long-term diet to follow.

If you want to try all three diets, it is actually possible and can help you lose weight. You can start by trying the Paleo diet first. Stop eating processed food and eat only natural ingredients for all meals. After a while switch over to the Atkins diet. Lastly, try the keto diet and restrict the carbohydrate content in your diet. This transition process can actually make it easier for someone who really wants to try the keto diet for weight loss. You get the benefit of all three diets in this way. If you combine exercise with this dietary change, you will lose weight and improve your health in no time.

Chapter Four:
Keto Diet Benefits and Side Effects

The keto diet is a very healthy and beneficial diet for those who follow it appropriately. In fact, it is not really like a diet at all but more of a lifestyle change. The keto lifestyle follows the eating habits that our ancestors evolved with and is thus natural for our bodies. Your body will not be exerted in an unnatural way that harms it. You won't have to curb hunger and cravings that are induced by other unhealthy diets.

• The first benefit that most people seek from this diet is weight loss and it really delivers results. The state of ketosis helps burn off the excess stored fat in all parts of the body over time. You will see the number on the scale go down but more importantly, you will see the shape of your body change with this loss in fat. This will give you a boost of confidence that you need to keep following a healthy lifestyle.

• The keto diet allows you to eat a lot of nutritious and good food. You don't need to eat bland tasteless foods that other fad diets recommend. In fact, all the butter and cheese that other diets restrict is what the keto diet recommends. Have you ever tried such a delicious diet before? You don't have to worry about counting calories for every meal and eating unsatisfyingly small portions. The food that was blamed for your weight is actually not the culprit at all. You can now enjoy these foods without feeling guilty about it.

•	The diet is not too restrictive like others that give you very few options for your meals. In fact, there are more than enough recipes for keto meals to eat something different every day. You won't get disheartened by the same boring meals while on this diet.

•	The state of ketosis will also make your mind more alert and focused. It is very beneficial for mental health and helps to function better since ketosis allows ketones to continually provide the brain with energy. The keto diet also helps to improve sleep patterns in your body.

•	Most people notice that they are not always as hungry as they used to be. Eating too often is a major cause for gaining weight and a carb-loaded diet usually causes this. In a keto diet, you will feel satisfied with your meals and tend not to eat more than two or three times a day at the most. Once you get used to the keto diet, you can start fasting and find that it is not too difficult for you anymore either.

- Another benefit of the keto diet is in regulating blood sugar levels. Excessive sugar or carbs in your diet raise blood sugar to an unhealthy level. Over time, more insulin is produced and your body becomes immune to high insulin levels. This can cause type two diabetes, which leads to many other conditions. Some of these symptoms include blindness, frequent urination, limb amputation, etc. The keto diet has been shown to help such people in regulating blood sugar. The lower levels of insulin also help to prevent some types of cancer cell growth; however, more research is being done on this latter aspect.

- Fatty liver disease is another condition that you should keep in mind. When you consume too much sugar or even alcohol, a lot of fat is collected in the liver. This can cause fatty liver disease, which is very harmful. The keto diet helps burn off the extra fat from the liver and other parts of the body. Excessive storage of fat is the main issue that keto deals with.

- Many people notice that their energy levels increase after the first few days of the ketogenic diet. Initially, the adaptation stage might make you feel dizzy and tired all the time. This can be avoided with a few things and after a while, it passes by itself anyway. Then you will see that you are much more alert and have more energy to go through all your activities.

•	The keto diet also helps to produce good HDL cholesterol and controlling LDL cholesterol. This will help prevent inflammation of the blood vessels. Too many carbohydrates in your diet increases triglycerides, which are reduced by higher fat consumption. Thus, the keto diet will help you in regulating your blood pressure preventing hardening of arteries and protecting against many heart conditions.

•	If you are suffering from a lot of acne breakouts, you will find that more often than not, carbohydrates make it worse. Too much insulin leads to the production of other acne-causing hormones. The ketogenic diet helps you cut down on these carbs and can reduce acne as well.

•	Some studies have also shown that the ketogenic diet helps control seizures in those suffering from epilepsy. Like cancer, this field is also still being worked on with no conclusive results as yet.

•	The ketogenic diet is also said to be beneficial for those with nervous system disorders such as Alzheimer's, Parkinson's, etc. The reasoning behind this is that the ketones help to promote brain health. This is why it also helps people who suffer from strong and frequent migraines by helping to reduce these.

- Polycystic Ovary Syndrome is found to be a condition many women suffer from these days. High levels of insulin in the body can cause this condition. Thus, a ketogenic diet will help to lower insulin levels and thus the risk of PCOS in women.

- Athletes who practice endurance sports also benefit from the ketogenic diet. This is because the muscle to fat ratio is improved and it provides the body more oxygen during such activities. Runners and cyclists need more energy for their sports and the keto diet helps to peak their performance.

- The keto diet also helps to keep uric acid levels in check, which are often the cause for gout or kidney stones. The keto diet raises uric acid levels temporarily when dehydrated but then reduces it.

- Starchy food like grains, potatoes, food laden with sugar, foods containing preservatives, etc. all increase the chance of acid reflux as well as heartburn. Reducing the carbs in your diet will help to deal with these symptoms.

Side Effects

There are some side effects that you might notice when you first start the keto diet. Unless you have some medical conditions, these side effects are usually not a cause for much concern. You might suffer from some constipation, indigestion or even low blood sugar.

One of the more major side effects might be acidosis or kidney stones due to the keto diet; however, these latter conditions do not usually occur. This is why we recommend a doctor's consultation to check if the ketogenic diet is appropriate for you. You should also go slowly as you make changes in your current diet since the body will be unaccustomed to it. This is especially the case for people who are too obese or have heart conditions.

There are three serious conditions that can cause side effects during a keto diet.

Hypoglycemia

The first is hypoglycemia. If you have hypoglycemia, you might feel dizzy, tired, extremely hungry and irritable while you adapt to the keto diet. These symptoms usually occur only during the first few weeks and subside later. You might also get flu-like symptoms like nausea, headaches and a runny nose. When you first cut out sugar, you might get intense sugar cravings that really challenge you to stick to the diet. This response will subside once the body gets used to producing ketones for energy.

Until your body adapts to the keto diet you will feel energy deficient. This is only for a short time until fats are used for energy. This causes the dizziness and drowsy feeling in the initial days. You will also notice that you don't have enough strength and feel weak during this keto-adaptation period. All these symptoms see drastic improvement when you get adapted to ketosis.

There are certain ways to deal with the effects of hypoglycemia. One is that you should eat every few hours to replenish energy in your body and prevent cravings. Also, drink liquids that have high mineral content like broths or electrolyte drinks. Stay hydrated all the time and add lots of salt to your food. Snack on foods like seaweed, cucumbers, and celery to curb hunger and get minerals replenished in your body. Also, add a magnesium supplement to your diet during this initial period.

HPA Axis Dysfunction

HPA axis dysfunction is another condition that can cause side effects during keto diets. This deals with the three glands hypothalamus, pituitary, and adrenal. These glands are usually responsible for regulation of stress responses in your body. During hypoglycemia, your brain will respond to starvation. The adrenals then release cortisol and this will signal for releasing of glucose stored in the body. This response causes quick burning up of glycogen stored in the body and hypoglycemia will reoccur. This HPA axis dysregulation causes related symptoms to reoccur. Disruption in sleep is also a common side effect due to this. It is because of the cortisol, which opposes the function of melatonin.

During HPA axis dysregulation, cortisol levels tend to fluctuate and the melatonin release at night is deterred. Cortisol is released during hypoglycemia and it causes the release of glycogen from all over the body. This stimulating hormone disrupts sleep at night if this response occurs then and can lead to insomnia or bad sleep patterns. Heart palpitations are also noticed in some people during the early keto-adaptation days. This is caused by hypoglycemia, a mineral imbalance and HPA axis issues. The abnormally high cortisol levels might cause cortisol resistance in the body. In response, more adrenaline is secreted and this causes an abnormal heart rhythm.

The mineral loss also leads to blood volume or pressure being reduced and this causes faster pumping of the heart. In order to take precautions against HPA axis dysfunction, there are certain steps you can take. You need to follow some strategies to maintain your blood sugar. Magnesium supplementation will also help to support the function of the HPA axis. Adaptogenic herbs are also said to be beneficial during the initial stage of keto-adaptation.

Mineral deficiencies can also be problematic during keto-adaptation. HPA axis dysfunction can cause excessive excretion of minerals through urine. These minerals and electrolytes are essential for water regulation and nerve conductivity functions. The HPA axis is responsible for cortisol and hydration regulation so it affects mineral retention or excretion.

One of the common symptoms of electrolyte imbalance is frequent urination. On a keto diet, insulin secretion decreases and sodium levels in urine increase. This sodium causes increased urination and is a common symptom of keto-adaptation. As the stored glycogen in the body is burnt, this also causes more water being sent to the urinary system. Urination helps get rid of toxins from the body and is a positive process; however, you need to supplement your body with the loss of minerals along with it. There are many side effects related to each mineral deficiency. Another sign of keto-adaptation is constipation and this occurs when the electrolyte balance is not maintained.

Water content plays an important role in this process. The change in microbiome in your stomach can also be a factor, which affects this process. Instead of constipation, some people might experience diarrhea. This is also dependent on the change in the microbiome of the stomach. Try taking a binding agent like activated charcoal or citrus pectin to solve this problem. Foods like eggs and nuts also affect the consistency of the stool. Muscle cramps are another early onset symptom experienced during a keto diet. Usually, it is also caused by an imbalance in minerals and poor hydration. You can avoid these problems using a few simple precautions as you begin the keto diet.

Firstly, drink a lot of water and mineral-rich liquids. Also, add generous amounts of high-quality salt to your food.

Keto breath

Keto breath is a common symptom or side effect of the keto diet. The ketones produced during ketosis occur in different forms. When the ketones are released with your breath, it is acetone and this is the keto breath. This usually wears off within a week or two of adaptation. Try using breath fresheners a few times in the day and ensure proper hydration.

All of these are symptoms that can easily be dealt with and even prevented with precaution. As long as your doctor says your health will support the keto diet, there is no reason to worry:

•   Stay well hydrated and add more minerals to your diet in order to prevent mineral imbalances. Add supplements like magnesium to provide your body what it needs.

•   If you feel light-headed or nauseous, monitor your blood pressure for a while as you start the keto diet. For those who take insulin or medication for lowering blood pressure, your dose needs to be reduced during the keto diet with a doctor's prescription. A blood glucose monitor will help to keep track of the changes in your body initially. Unless it is too abnormal, you don't have reason to worry.

•	Taking exogenous ketones will also be beneficial in helping the body adapt to the increased ketosis.

•	Increase the frequency of your meals throughout the day to deal with hypoglycemia. Add more salt to your food as well.

•	Organic broths will help you a lot during the initial keto diet adaptation. These add more minerals and amino acids to your diet.

Chapter Five:
Foods to Eat and Foods to Avoid

You should have a general idea about the concept of a ketogenic diet by now. You probably want to get started and begin your keto diet immediately; you should first clear out all non-ketogenic foods from your pantry or kitchen first. Get rid of any unhealthy processed and ready-to-eat foods. You can make a list of the foods that are ketogenic and non-ketogenic before you go shopping. It can actually be quite frustrating trying to figure out what you should and should not buy while you are on a diet. I will help you get started with this.

Foods to Avoid

• Grains in the form of wheat, barley, rye, sorghum, corn, bulgur, oats, quinoa, amaranth, rice, millet, buckwheat, etc. Avoid any bread, pasta, cookies or even pizza crusts made from these grains. All grains should be avoided on a low carb diet since they will slow the weight loss process.

• Beans or legumes in the form of kidney beans, pinto beans, green peas, lima beans, fava beans, black beans, chickpeas, lentils, white beans, cannellini beans, etc. The high starch content in beans makes them unsuitable for a keto diet.

• Fruits like bananas, oranges, pineapples, papaya, grapes, mangoes, apples and tangerines. Avoid any fruit syrups, packaged fruit juices, fruit concentrates or even dried fruits. Everyone says fruits are healthy but they are not keto friendly. This is because of the high sugar and carb content in them.

• Starchy vegetables like sweet potatoes, peas, yams, corn, yucca, cherry tomatoes, carrots or parsnips. These high carb containing vegetables are not suitable for a keto diet.

• Sugar in the form of honey, agave nectar, cane sugar, turbinado sugar, maple syrup, high fructose corn syrup, etc. Sugar should be avoided in any form.

• Milk and low-fat dairy products like shredded cheese, fat-free butter, low-fat cream cheese, skim milk, low fat whipped cream, low-fat yogurt, etc.

• Factory farmed animal products like grain fed meats, canned meat, beef jerky, packaged sausages, bacon, chicken nuggets, fish sticks, corned beef, salami, hot dogs or factory farmed fish.

• Unhealthy fats in the form of canola oil, safflower oil, sunflower oil, grapeseed oil, peanut oil, corn oil or soybean oil.

•   Alcohol like beers, wines, cocktails, flavored liquors.

•   Sweetened beverages like sodas, diet sodas, juices, tea or coffee with sweeteners, milk products with sweeteners, etc.

•   Packaged cookies and cakes or candies and ice creams. Avoid almond milk products and foods with gelatin.

•   Avoid any artificial sweeteners like Equal, Splenda, Saccharin, Sucralose, etc.

•   Don't eat fast food from any restaurants.

•   Don't eat margarine instead of butter. It is an industrially modified form of butter with too much omega 6 fat and has no nutritional benefit.

•   Avoid condiments with any of the unhealthy oils or added sugars or labeled low fat.

Foods to eat

•   Eat unprocessed meat that is low in carbs and thus keto friendly. Any organic or grass-fed meat is usually appropriate for a keto meal. Remember not to overeat meat since your protein intake has to be moderate and fat intake increased. If you eat too much meat, you eat too much protein and this gets converted to glucose for energy

•   Fish and seafood are very keto friendly. Try to get fresh and wild fish and avoid breeding fish. Fatty fish like salmon are a good bet.

•   Eggs cooked in any form are keto friendly. Try to acquire organic eggs.

•   Eat vegetables that grow above ground and avoid root vegetables like potato. Leafy and green vegetables are the best. You can also add more cauliflower, zucchini, broccoli cabbage, and avocado to your diet. Cook them in some fatty butter or oil to make it keto friendly. Add more vegetables to your plate to make up for the grains you will avoid on keto.

•   High-fat dairy like butter, cheese, heavy cream, etc is good for a keto diet. The more fat the better; however, try to avoid milk since milk sugar adds up. Always eat full-fat yogurt and keep away from the low-fat kind.

•   Nuts are great to eat but they should be eaten in moderation. It is easy to overeat nuts while snacking. Cashews should be eaten minimally since they contain a lot of carbs.

•   Low-sugar fruits like berries are keto friendly in moderate amounts. Berries are a good substitute for sugary desserts. Add some full-fat whipping cream to a bowl of berries for your sweet fix.

•   Coffee is fine if you don't add sugar. If you need milk it should be very little and use full-fat cream.

•   Water is the best liquid you can hydrate with. You can add natural flavoring to your water like cucumbers, lemons, etc to drink more often.

•   Tea of any kind is healthy but don't add sugar. Certain teas like green tea or oolong tea actually help to lose weight faster on the keto diet.

•   Bone broth is highly recommended on a keto diet. It contains a lot of nutrients and electrolytes and is very simple to prepare. Adding a bit of butter to it makes it taste better and is keto effective as well.

•   If you want alcohol for a special occasion, try dry wine or any alcohol without sugar and only have a glass.

• Dark chocolate can be a treat for a cheat day. Buy dark chocolate with high amounts of cocoa. You can use this to prepare keto desserts as well.

Fats and oils are usually avoided or prohibited on all other diets; however, here we encourage adding these to your diet. Fats can be very helpful in losing weight as long as they are the right kind of fats. A keto diet guides you in consuming more healthy fat in your diet every single day. The fats that you need to avoid are in potato chips, cookies, and other processed snacks. You need more of the monosaturated fats like those in butter, tuna, avocado, etc. Omega 3 is another nutrient that you need to add to your diet. Fish is the best source for this but supplements are also available in most stores. Hydrogenated fats should also be removed from your diet. These are usually in the form of vegetable oils. Increase your fatty oil intakes with food like chicken fat, beef tallow, olive oil, butter, and avocado.

Proteins in a moderate amount is required in a ketogenic diet. They should be consumed in lower amounts than fat content but more than carbs. Proteins help to prevent hunger and increase energy levels. For protein sources, look for organic and grass-fed options. If you like eggs, they are keto friendly with lots of protein but try to buy free range eggs. Fish, red meat, poultry, and shellfish are healthy sources of protein.

A lot of people don't enjoy eating vegetables but you need to remember that they are an essential part of any diet. Vegetables are filled with nutrients that other sources can't always provide you. Those that grow above ground are more keto friendly than the vegetables that grow below ground. Leafy greens are a very good addition to your diet and actually help you feel full faster. Try to buy fresh vegetables that are organically grown and free from pesticides. If you want to go the extra mile and like gardening, grow some of your own vegetables. This way, you know exactly what goes in your stomach without worrying about chemicals. You can't load up your plate with every vegetable since some are quite high in starch and sugar. The most ketogenic vegetables are celery, asparagus, mushrooms, onions, broccoli, avocado, and romaine lettuce.

While shopping for ketogenic foods, beware of foods that are labeled low carb or keto friendly. Don't trust commercial products at face value and read the list of ingredients provided on the label. There are always hidden ingredients that you really need to avoid. Packaged foods are usually unhealthy and don't help to lose weight no matter what the label says. These days there are more products being shelved labeled as low fat, low carb, diet, ketogenic, etc; however, most of these have hidden ingredients that will harm you in the long run. Any food with artificial sweeteners, additives, alcohol etc. should be avoided. Remember, you cannot replace real sugar with marketed fake sugar. Also, beware of labels since companies often lie to sell their product.

Raw full-fat dairy products are also ketogenic. Heavy whipping cream, cheese, sour cream, etc. are all good sources of vitamin D and proteins in your diet. They should not be consumed in excess but can be added to your diet.

Nuts are a very healthy snack to keep around as long as you can control yourself from eating too much. They are packed with protein and nutrients and a small amount is more than enough. Roasting nuts are a good way to get rid of any pesticides or additives that might be harmful. Amongst nuts, avoid eating too many cashews and also avoid peanuts, which are a part of legumes. Peanuts are not ketogenic friendly. If you buy packaged nuts, buy the unsalted variety. Healthy options for nuts include pistachio, walnuts, sunflower seeds, macadamias, and almonds. More than a handful of nuts every day is not recommended. A little every day will give you a good source of omega 6 and protein.

While following the ketogenic diet, one of the most common symptoms or side effects is dehydration. This diet has a diuretic effect that can be harmful if you do not hydrate your body sufficiently. This is more prominent in the first few weeks of starting the keto diet. Always carry a bottle of water with you during this time. This will keep your body cool and hydrated. You need to remember to drink twice the usual amount of water during the first few days. Dehydration can have detrimental effects on your body in the long run. Other than water you can also drink herbal teas, unsweetened tea or coffee, and fruit water.

Your best bet during a keto diet, or any healthy diet, is to eat real wholesome food and home-cooked meals. The more minimally processed your ingredients are, the better it is for you. Ideally, buy raw fresh ingredients and nothing canned or labeled. Also, remember that it is a low carb diet and not a no carb diet. You just need to keep the carbs to a minimum in your daily intake. The diet does not have to be stressful for you. You can eat without staying hungry and still lose weight while following the keto diet. If you follow the diet properly, it will have a very beneficial effect on your health and a positive impact on your life. Eating right is very important.

How To Get Started?

Now that you know what the keto diet is and the foods you can or cannot eat, you can get started. Many people find it hard to get started with a new diet, especially when there are too many rules and instructions involved. Each diet tells you something different to do and it can be confusing. The ketogenic diet is comparatively very easy to follow. The basic rule of thumb is to avoid factory-processed food and eat wholesome meals.

Any packaged and commercially sold food

items will have many hidden ingredients that you aren't really aware of. These will include sugars, preservatives, additives, etc. that are all unhealthy for you. A glass of soda will usually have more sugar than your required dietary allowance and more often than not you tend to drink a few glasses a day. Sugar itself is a very bad ingredient in your diet and should be cut off as soon as possible. Processed foods with sugar are one of the main causes of gaining weight and lead to obesity. Even if what you buy is not sweet, sugar might be an ingredient in it in another form.

Check the labels for ingredients every time you buy a processed product. You might not realize it but pizza also contains sugar. Even in labels, sugar is written in different names. There are hundreds of products on the market with sugar in them, so it is not surprising that obesity has been increasing at an alarming rate each year. The keto diet just helps you understand what is healthy and unhealthy for your body so that you can make better choices. While other diets will tell you to lose weight by not eating much, the keto diet will help you eat and still lose weight.

The easiest way to avoid hidden ingredients like colorants, preservatives, and sugars is to buy raw ingredients or even grow them. The list of foods to avoid and eat will be helpful during your grocery trips. Farmers markets are a good way to buy organic produce that is healthy for you. Avoid ingredients that are high in carbs like potatoes even if they're your favorite vegetable. If you always eat bread or some grain with your regular meals, you need to remember that they will only make you gain weight. It is crucial to stop eating more than 20gm of carbs every day while you follow a ketogenic diet. If you have foods with too many carbs, your body will find it harder to go into the state of ketosis and the diet will not work for you. Replace these parts of your meal with healthier substitutes. If you really need bread then use almond flour to bake healthier bread. Healthier alternatives can be found for many of the foods that are not keto friendly. The oils that you use for cooking or as salad dressing should also be keto friendly. They will still taste just as good. Cooking with butter can actually make most dishes taste richer and better. Who knew butter was good for you? Olive oil and walnut oil are much healthier than most seed oils that you usually use.

To get started there are a few examples of meals that you can prepare on the keto diet after this chapter. This will give you a head start but there are many more recipes that you can try each and every day while you stay on the ketogenic routine. The first step is to be determined that you want to achieve a certain goal. Get rid of any food in the house that is not keto friendly. Buy all the healthy ingredients recommended above and stock your pantry. Start trying out new recipes to make it a fun transition.

The first week or so can be a little difficult if you notice some side effects from your keto diet.

Before you begin, get a check-up and ask your doctor if the diet is suitable for your body. If you get their approval, the common side effects are just temporary and will pass. You can even take precautions and avoid symptoms like dizziness, dehydration, etc. If something seems too unnatural for you, just consult your doctor again. A few supplements and a lot of water usually do the trick. You need to persevere through the initial adaptation stage and let your body get used to the new diet. Soon your system will get used to the ketogenic foods and act accordingly. As your body starts going into ketosis, you will start burning stored fat and lose weight. Usually, your body will help you lose weight until it reaches an appropriate number and then maintain it.

If you feel like you are losing too much weight, you can always adjust your diet accordingly. For those who exercise regularly, it is not necessary to load up on carbs. Fats will also provide you with the energy you need. If your activities are too intense you can add a little more carbohydrates if your trainer recommends it. The keto diet is good enough regardless of what else you do.

You need to remember that everyone's body is different and will react differently. The diet might work better for some people and help them lose weight faster. The process might be slower for others. It will just depend on the individual and neither is right or wrong. The keto diet will work slowly and help you achieve a healthy weight and help you maintain it. It is not a fad diet that will make you skinny through starvation. If you don't notice any changes over a long time, you might not be following the diet properly. It is important to reduce carbs, keep proteins moderate, eat a lot of fat and cut out all manufactured products. The diet will help you if you help yourself. A cheat day is allowed once in a while but if you do it too often, the diet won't work for you. If you really want to lose weight, I recommend avoiding cheat days until you've at least reached your goal weight. Eating junk food once in a while can also shake your resolve to stick to the diet and all your effort will be in vain. Stick to the list of keto foods and watch it work for you. Adding some regular exercise will just help it work better for you but is not a compulsory requirement in the keto diet.

Overview of the Keto Diet

These are the important points to keep in mind when you start the keto diet so that you can effectively push your system into ketosis.

- First, you have to make sure you restrict your carbohydrate intake to around 20g or less per day. The diet is strictly low carb or it won't work for you. You don't need to cut out fiber since it is required for your body, but reducing carbs in your diet will make a huge difference and help you lose weight through ketosis.

- You also have to control your protein intake and keep it moderate - but more - compared to your carbohydrate intake. Usually, you should eat at least 1-2g of protein per kg of your body weight every day. Keep the amount moderate since protein can also be converted to glucose by the body and this will hinder the process of ketosis.

- The most important part of the keto diet is including a lot of fat in it. Fat will help you eat a full meal and stay satisfied till your next meal. A carb-loaded diet gets burned off easily and leads to hunger and binge eating. Eating more fats will be a more sustainable way to check your eating habits and force your body to go into ketosis. This will help you lose a lot of weight.

- Don't develop a habit of snacking too often. There are many keto snacks that are available to suit your diet but it is better to stick to the main meals and only snack a day at the most. Eating unnecessarily and untimely is a bad habit that will slow down the ketosis and also make you gain weight. Snacking is one of the worst habits of the modern-day diet and is caused due to the thousands of products easily available to binge on around us. Don't buy a ton of snacks when you visit the supermarket because this just makes it harder to resist at home.

- Stay hydrated throughout the day whether you are on the diet or not. When you first start keto dieting, increase your water intake a little more than usual.

- Add exercise to your daily routine to burn off fat faster. Physical activity has many benefits for the body; it will help you stay fit, promotes longevity and helps prevent many diseases.

- Try adding intermittent fasting to your routine after a while. This is effective in increasing ketones in the body and accelerating the process of weight loss during ketosis.

- Also, make sure you get sufficient sleep. A good night's rest is essential for the body to maintain good health. Lack of sleep can cause many issues like blood sugar imbalance, increased stress hormone secretion, etc. Sleep deprivation will leave you feeling tired and unwell the next day. Bad sleeping patterns also slow down ketosis and promote bad eating habits. Midnight snacks might sound fun but are not a healthy choice especially if you want to lose weight.

- Unless you are an athlete or take part in very demanding sports, you generally don't need any supplements during the ketogenic diet. Adding supplements is not recommended unless necessary. It's better not to waste a ton of money on any products that claim to increase the rate of your weight loss either. Just stick to the diet and it will work for you.

- Remember to consult your doctor to see if there are any underlying medical conditions that make the keto diet unsuitable for you. Don't rush into any diet at the risk of your health. Different things might work for different people. As long as they give you a positive affirmation, you can get started with the keto diet and start losing weight as soon as possible.

If you want to check whether your body has entered the state of ketosis, there are certain tools that help you measure it:

- The first is urine strips that are easily available and an affordable option. You just have to dip the urine strip in your urine. Color change is used to indicate the presence of ketones in your urine. If the reading on the strip is high or the darkest color then you will know that your body is undergoing ketosis.

- Ketone breath analyzers are another option. These are much more expensive than urine strips but are reusable unlike the latter. There is no precise marker for the level of ketones in your breath but the analyzer helps to check if they are present or not using a color code.

- The most expensive tool to measure ketosis is the blood ketone meter. This is the most accurate tool to measure the presence and level of ketones in your blood. The only disadvantage of blood ketone meters is that they are extremely expensive; however, there are cheaper tests available these days to make it more feasible.

Any of the above tools can be used if you want to check the presence of ketones in your body and learn if the ketosis process has begun. This can be an encouraging way to stick to the diet and continue ketosis for losing weight.

Another thing that you can take note of is how to know if your body is at the optimal level of ketosis. Blood ketone meters have very specific markings that will help you out with this aspect. If the level shows itself to be below 0.5 mmol/l then this is not ketosis, but you are getting close to it; however, this low level will never help you burn fat in your body. In the initial stage, you might find the level between 0.5 mmol/l and 1.5 mmol/l. This is a lower level of ketosis which is beneficial but still not optimal for the kind of results you want. Optimal ketosis occurs between 1.5 and 3 mmol/l. This level is recommended the most for seeing the maximum results from ketosis.

At this level, ketosis will result in burning a lot of the excess fat stored in your body and speed up the process of weight loss.

You will also see better mental and physical

performance when you enter this state. If your blood ketone level if more than 3 mmol/l then it is higher than recommended. It won't show you any special results compared to the optimal level so don't try to push your body to this state. This level usually indicates that you have not been eating enough and is called starvation ketosis. Those who suffer from diabetes type 1 often experience this due to lack of insulin. The most dangerous level is 8-10 mmol/l, which is very uncommon but is a bad ketone count. It is associated with diabetes Type I most of the time and has severe symptoms like nausea, abdominal pain, confusion, etc. You will feel very unwell if your ketone levels are this high and it can even be fatal so get immediate medical attention.

The blood ketone meter can be a very useful tool in checking if you are going about your diet in the right way. Don't over-do it and try to push your body into ketosis slowly. Also, don't try to starve yourself to achieve weight loss faster. This does not work with the ketogenic diet and is against its principles. Allow the diet to be beneficial for you by following all its guidelines.

Achieving the optimal blood ketone level is your aim and you should work to maintain it when you get there. Don't assume that higher ketone levels will help you burn even more fat and lose weight. The cost of weight loss should not be your health. Your goal is to lose weight in a healthy way to improve the mental and physical state of your body. If you follow the ketogenic diet in the right way, you will definitely achieve this.

Chapter Six:
*5 Examples of Meals/Recipes Allowed on the
Ketogenic Diet*

Here I will give you examples of some recipes that you can try when you start the ketogenic diet. There are many dishes that you can make with keto ingredients that will be healthy for you. Throughout the day on a keto diet, don't skip meals and when you first start, try to eat small meals 4 to 5 times a day. Drink water or any keto-friendly beverage multiple times a day to prevent dehydration. Don't drink any packaged juices or fizzy drinks, which have no nutritional value. If you want a small snack in-between meals, have a cup of full-fat yogurt with some berries or maybe just a small cup of fruit. A handful of nuts are also a good choice but don't overeat these or fruits which can contain a lot of sugar.

Prepare meals according to your convenience and try to eat at home as often as possible; however, as you read on you will see that I have shown you how to stay on the keto diet even when you go out to restaurants or go traveling. Some days you can just have a small meal with one dish and on others, you can prepare a whole spread just for yourself. Just try to keep a watch on how much you eat if you want to lose weight and not gain it. The best part of the keto diet is how it allows you to eat so much good food without stressing about limits. You can trust your instincts when it comes to the right quantity of food to eat as long as all the ingredients are ketogenic.

Breakfast

Let's start with breakfast. You can start your day with some tea or coffee depending on your preference. Don't add any sugar or artificial sweetener to these. Full fat milk or cream is allowed on a keto diet. Start hydrating yourself from the beginning of the day. Try to have at least 8-10 glasses of water in the day. This will prevent dehydration and flush out toxins from your body. If you don't have time to make a full breakfast spread, just grab some fruit or yogurt. On holidays, make the effort to eat a more elaborate spread that will really satisfy you. The keto diet really allows you to enjoy the food that others tell you not to.

Do you love pancakes? Well, you can make your own keto friendly breakfast pancakes using this recipe. There's no need to stress out about what to eat early in the morning. There are a ton of keto friendly breakfast recipes that you can quickly whip up in the morning. Some of them are indicated on the next page.

Keto Blueberry Pancakes

Ingredients:
3 eggs
2 oz. cream cheese
2 oz, butter (melted)
1/3 cup almond flour
1/3 cup oat fiber
1 tsp baking powder
Lemon zest
A pinch of salt
2 oz. blueberries

Method:

1.   Take a mixing bowl and break the eggs into it. Add the cream cheese and melted butter to this and whisk well.
2.   After the above mixture is thoroughly mixed, add the remaining ingredients into this batter other than the blueberries. Mix these properly into the batter and let it sit for a while.
3.   Place a non-stick pan over medium heat. Pour a little batter into it depending on the size of the pancakes you want. Add the blueberries when you add the batter to the pan. Fry both sides for a while and remove. Repeat this till the batter is over.
4.   Enjoy the pancakes with some full fat whipped cream. Double the amount of ingredients according to the number of people you want to serve.

Keto Coconut Pancakes

Ingredients:
3 eggs
1/3 cup coconut flour
1/3 cup coconut milk
1 tbsp coconut oil
A pinch of salt
½ tsp baking powder
Butter

Method:

1.   Take two bowls. Break the eggs and separate the whites into one bowl and yolks into the other bowl.
2.   Whisk the egg whites till frothy and add a pinch of salt to it. Once you see peaks form, keep this bowl aside.
3.   Whisk the egg yolks in the other bowl and add the coconut milk and coconut oil to this. Mix it well.
4.   Add baking powder and the coconut flour into the yolk batter. Mix it all in till you get a smooth consistency.
5.   Pour the whisked egg whites into the above batter. Mix well and keep it aside for a couple of minutes.
6.   Place a non-stick pan on medium heat. Add a spoon of butter and use a ladle to pour some pancake mixture into this. Fry each side till cooked

through. Don't press the pancake down or it won't be fluffy.

7.	Repeat the procedure for the entire batter and serve the hot coconut pancakes for breakfast.

Lunch

Lunch is another important meal of the day. There are a lot of keto lunch recipes that can be made quickly or take time depending on your convenience. You can whip up a quick but delicious salad with leafy greens, shredded meat, and healthy dressing. Add some poached eggs or mashed avocado to these. You can even make a smoothie and keep it prepared for days when you're short on time.

Lunch recipes: Lunch on a keto diet does not consist of a tasteless salad or some blended vegetables. You can easily prepare a delicious meal that is even better than what you normally eat. Some recipes can be found on the following page.

Keto frittata

Ingredients:
15 oz ground breakfast sausage
2 bell peppers
14 eggs
1 cup sour cream
Pinch of Himalayan salt
1 tsp black pepper
3 tsp butter
3 oz cheddar

Method:

1.   Keep your oven preheated to 360F.
2.   Crack all the eggs into a bowl and pour these into the blender with the sour cream. Add some salt and pepper to it. Blend this thoroughly and keep it aside.
3.   Place a non-stick pan on medium heat. Once it is heated add some butter to it.
4.   Cut the bell peppers into slices and fry these in the pan. Cook for a few minutes till they are brown and then remove from the pan.
5.   Now fry the breakfast sausage till it is properly brown and cooked. Press and flatten the meat into the pan. Add the peppers to this meat.
6.   Add the eggs on top of the meat and place it in the oven to bake for 25-30 minutes. Take it out at the halfway point and add the cheese on top. Then bake till everything is well cooked and the

cheese is melted well on the frittata.
7.	Take it out of the oven and enjoy a healthy lunch.

Dinner

Most people have time to prepare a proper dinner even if lunch was skipped or was a quick meal. Take your time to prepare and enjoy a healthy keto dinner. You can follow recipes or just try some experimentations depending on your taste.

Dinner recipe: A hearty and healthy meal makes everyone feel good. With keto recipes, you can cook delicious food, eat until you're full and still lose weight. This meatloaf recipe is the perfect way to kick-start your keto diet.

Keto Meatloaf
Ingredients:
2 tbsp beef tallow
2 small onions
4 cloves garlic
4 pounds ground beef
4 eggs
3 tbsp oregano
3 tsp salt
½ tsp pepper
1 cup low carb marinara sauce
½ cup almond flour

Method:

1.   Keep your oven preheated to 340F.
2.   Use a non-stick pan and place it on high heat. Dice the onion and garlic and saute them till cooked. Keep it aside for a while.
3.   Take a large bowl and mix the onion and garlic with the rest of the ingredients. Don't add the marinara sauce to this. Mix the rest of it well together with your hands.
4.   Now press this mixture into a lined loaf tin. Make sure there aren't any air bubbles and keep the top smooth. Bake this for 40-50 minutes.
5.   Pour out some of the extra juice when you take the tin out. Add the marinara sauce on top of the meatloaf. Then place it to bake for 10 more minutes.
6.   Take it out of the oven once it is done and let it sit for a while. Then slice and enjoy your delicious keto meatloaf with your family.

Keto dessert

Who says you can't enjoy dessert on a keto diet? There are always healthy alternatives that can still satisfy your sweet tooth. The trick is to choose the right ingredients and not over-do it. This recipe is perfect for anyone with a weakness for brownies.

Keto Brownies

Ingredients:
1 cup coconut almond butter
1 cup dark chocolate chips
1 cup avocado, mashed
2 tbsp coconut oil
4 tbsp chocolate stevia
6 tbsp cocoa powder

Method:

1.   Preheat your oven to 340F.
2.   Grease a baking pan with some coconut oil.
3.   Take a food blender and pour the coconut oil, cocoa powder, nut butter, avocado and stevia into it. Now blend into a smooth mixture.
4.   Pour the blended batter into a bowl and add the chocolate chips to it. Fold them into the batter and then spread it into the baking tin evenly.
5.   Place the tin into the oven for around 20 minutes until the brownie is done. Now take it out, let it cool, cut and serve.

Do any of the recipes given here sound boring or tasteless? I'm sure you're actually looking forward to trying them. They are all delicious dishes that will make you appreciate how versatile the meals of a keto diet are. You can find many more sources for keto recipes in cookbooks or online and try them out every day.

A ketogenic eater probably has more meals available to him/her than anyone on any other diet, but this doesn't mean you have free reign to eat as much and as often as you please. There is a limit to how much food your body actually needs. Just eat enough to satisfy your hunger but don't try to fill a pit where your stomach is. Snacking is actually one of the easiest ways to gain weight so watch what you eat in between meals. This is why we recommend eating a full meal at the right time. A healthy keto meal will easily get your body accustomed to preventing cravings.

We also recommend trying to meal prep each week so that you don't spend too much time preparing meals. Meal prepping once a week will save you a lot of time and also help you to avoid any stress about making keto meals. This way you can easily stay on track with your keto diet. Over time, you will get used to it and won't even need a list to tell you what is keto-friendly and what isn't. You can even create your own keto recipes to share with others.

Chapter Seven:
Tracking Macros and Counting Calories

Let's first take a look at macros. Macros or macronutrients are the larger nutrient class that your body uses for energy. It includes protein, fats, and carbohydrates and these are referred to as macros. Micronutrients are required in small amounts in our body but these macros are required in larger amounts to provide the appropriate energy.

A keto diet aims to burn fat instead of carbs for energy in the body. This is achieved by limiting your intake of carbs. This is why you might find it useful to track your macro consumption when you start the keto diet. You need to learn to consume fewer carbs on a low-carb keto diet. Usually, it is recommended to keep it to a maximum of 20gm carbs each day. This is essential for pushing the body into ketosis.

Tracking your macros will help you to ensure that you are eating in a way that your body enters the ketosis state and burns stored fat. You need to see to it that fats constitute 70% of your diet, carbs 5% and proteins 25%. This is the ideal distribution of macros for a keto diet. In order to keep track of these, you can easily choose from an array of keto apps available on smartphones these days. All you need to enter is the basic date of your meals and they will help you keep track of what you are eating. They also factor in any additional exercise that you do to help you lose weight. Many of these have features to remind you to eat frequent meals, drink water, etc. Once you start using these trackers you can see how simple it is to stay on track with your keto diet. You can also find many keto recipes on these to help you cook the right kind of meals.

Like I said before, a keto diet does not require counting calories for every meal; however, if you really want to stick to a strict diet and prefer it, you can keep track of your calories quite easily. Counting calories can actually be helpful while you try to lose weight because it gives you a clear picture of what you are putting into your body. It also makes it easier for you to notice when you might be overeating. On a ketogenic diet, calorie counting should only be used as a tool to help you out. Don't get stressed or obsess over this aspect since it isn't essential as long as you stick to the guidelines for a ketogenic lifestyle.

Calorie counting will help you to keep track of how much energy you are putting into your body and how much you really need. This will depend on an individual's activities, metabolic rate, general health, etc. All these will affect how much energy you spend in a day and also help you determine how much you need to consume.

In a ketogenic diet, you should consume fewer calories than your body regularly needs. In this way, it will use the stored energy to make up for the calories you did not consume. For instance, if you need 2000 calories per day for all your activities, you should consume around 1500 calories. Your body will then use fat to get the 500 calories worth of energy. This way you can also approximately track how many calories your body burns every day and week; however, you need to remember that there is no fixed equation or result for this. It is just a basic concept that you can use while counting calories during your diet.

Calories do matter but it is not important to keep looking at them. Trust your body and eat enough to satiate your hunger but not overeat. If you count calories and keep yourself hungry, you will just end up binge eating later. Overeating is always unhealthy so that is a basic aspect that applies no matter what diet you are on. Just focus on eating the right food in the appropriate amounts and your body will work to keep you healthy by itself. Calorie counting will not determine your process. Just limiting your calories to a certain extent will help to burn stored fat and assist in your weight loss, nothing more.

Intermittent Fasting and the Keto Diet

Have you heard of intermittent fasting? It is one of the most popular methods to lose weight these days and for good reason. Fasting has long been practiced in many cultures as a part of rituals or ceremonies. In general, fasting is a good way to give your body a break and detoxify. Similar to the keto diet, intermittent fasting helps balance blood glucose levels, improving food habits, losing weight, etc.

This is why if you try intermittent fasting with your keto diet, it might give you better results. Both these diets are sustainable for a long time and instill good habits in you. Once you get the hang of it, you get used to practicing a better food lifestyle in the long run and that should be your aim. Don't try to lose weight with fad diets that give you temporary results. Most of these only help you lose water weight or cause you to relapse into overeating out of hunger.

Starving yourself can be very detrimental for your health and also lead to eating disorders; however, fasting is not the same as starving yourself. Fasting is a method where you practice self-discipline and give your body a break from food. It is actually not essential to eat a lot all the time. During fasting days, your body can easily use stored fat for energy and still function normally. You just need to stay hydrated and not think too much about it.

As you know, the keto diet helps you to burn stored fat by restricting consumption of excess carbohydrates. This is why it is effective in losing weight. You also get to eat all your meals so this means that you don't have untimely cravings on this diet. These factors in themselves help you to lose weight quite quickly; however, if you add intermittent fasting to this routine, you might see even better results.

Intermittent fasting is a process, which limits

the number of hours you eat and don't eat. A fasting plan can be created according to an individual's health and needs. Usually, you can choose to fast for anything from 15 hours to a whole 24 hours. Once you finish this fasting period, you can eat as you normally do. You just need to remember not to binge out in an effort to make up for the fasting duration. If you are also on a keto diet, then after your fasting period is over, eat keto meals. That is the only difference. Since you are getting your body used to eating lower amounts of carbohydrates, you will see that you experience fewer instances of cravings than before. This is because carbs get burnt quickly and usually end up leaving you feeling hungry again. The fats in a keto diet, on the other hand, take a longer time to burn and are thus successful in keeping you full for a long time.

There are many advantages to combining intermittent fasting with a ketogenic diet.

• Firstly, you will see that ketosis works at a faster rate than normal or if you just used one of these methods. If you are on a normal diet while fasting, your body will just burn all the carbs first, then the proteins and only burn fats in the end. This means very little fat will be burnt during the fasting period; however, if you are on a keto diet, you will consume minimal carbs. Hence, on a fasting day, these few carbs and proteins get burnt fast and your body will spend the rest of the time burning the fats in your body. Thus, your body achieves the state of ketosis faster when you are on an intermittent fasting routine and keto diet at the same time.

• Secondly, both these methods have shown to help stabilize blood sugar levels in the body. If you are on a high carb diet, your glucose levels will go low very quickly and make you hungry again. This leads to binge eating and thus weight gain. On a low carb diet along with fasting, your blood sugar is more stabilized and you see an improvement in focus, memory, etc.

• Another benefit of this combination is that your body will absorb vitamins and minerals better compared to before. Studies were conducted which showed that those who worked out after a fasting period were able to absorb nutrients more effectively. Thus, fasting might help to improve your body's nutrient absorption and also improve your overall health.

• Perhaps the most advantageous factor is that intermittent fasting and keto dieting can help you to lose weight in a faster way together than individually. When you add fasting to your routine, it gives your body more time to burn fat and it gets used to continuing ketosis for a longer time. Keto dieting itself will help your body learn to use stored fat from the body for energy and lose weight. If you are also fasting, your body will burn more fat to acquire energy and thus you lose weight in a much faster way.

• Combining keto dieting with intermittent fasting also helps your body to learn to avoid binge eating and cravings. The keto diet will help to prevent hunger and unhealthy cravings. Fats are much more fulfilling than carbs so this diet keeps you satisfied for longer periods of time. This means you won't be reaching for snacks every hour and craving unhealthy carbs to fill your stomach. When you start getting used to intermittent fasting, your body and mind will learn not to obsess over food but enjoy it and utilize it for energy.

• Detoxification is another benefit that you will experience during this process. A state of detoxification is achieved when you are not eating. Your body starts using and eliminating any unwanted elements in your body and helps you to get rid of them. In this way, you detoxify the body and help it stay healthy. Combining a keto diet with fasting also helps you to accelerate this process and reduce the risk of diseases like diabetes and heart conditions.

• Fasting is a very beneficial practice for mental health. Especially in Buddhist culture, it is a commonly practiced process. You can focus on other things and also see that you are more alert during your fasting period. Ketosis is also beneficial for your brain and mental health. Practicing both of these at the same time will reduce your risk of many conditions like Alzheimer's, Parkinson's disease, depression, strokes, etc. This is why you should consider it not just for the weight loss benefits.

You can easily understand why many people try to implement intermittent fasting with ketogenic diets. You can try it for yourself to see if you get the results they have claimed. If you find it too hard to start both at the same time, just begin with keto dieting for a month or so. Once you get used to it, start implementing a routine of intermittent fasting as well. The advantage of intermittent fasting is that it can be flexible. You can create a plan that suits you personally. If you are a compulsive eater and find it hard to stay hungry for a long time, you can start with skipping a meal, then another and then try a 15-hour fasting period for one day.

After 3 days, try it again and add a few hours to this if it wasn't too difficult. In this way, you can lead yourself to a full 24 hours of fasting. Remember not to fast for 2 days in a row. Your fasting should just be a break in a routine. Over time your body will get used to fasting and you can start fasting for at least three days a week. This combined with the ketogenic diet will help you lose a lot of weight quickly. It is easy to learn to build up a habit of intermittent fasting. Your body will just get used to it over time. It will start performing ketosis faster during fasting periods and help to burn up the unwanted stored fat in your body. This will help you see very prominent changes in your body over time.

Remember to drink a lot of water on all days of fasting or non-fasting. Don't let your body get dehydrated at any point. Also, as you implement intermittent fasting, you can keep changing your routine. Fast for longer periods when you can and just do it for a few hours on days where you need more energy. Adjust it to your lifestyle and don't let it overwhelm you. A different approach will suit a different person. You need to experiment and find what is appropriate for you.

While you are fasting or just following the keto diet, keep yourself busy. Don't stay idle and think too much about not eating or what you are eating or counting calories. These methods are meant to improve your way of life and not stress you out or affect you negatively. Many fad diets end up affecting the physical and mental health of people. They think that eating will make them gain weight so they avoid meals, vomit after meals and keep track of every single thing they consume. This can be very detrimental to their health and lead to many conditions.

Starvation can also be fatal for people with such eating disorders. This is where the keto diet is much better and so is the intermittent fasting method. You can enjoy your meals and still be assured that you will lose the excess weight that you previously gained. There is no focus on calories and skipping meals in a way that makes your body unhealthy. Remember, your goal is not just a particular number on the scale. You need to feel and look better at the same time no matter what that size of your body is.

No diet will be perfect for everyone. You just need to try and find what is effective and healthy for you. Consult a doctor to find what is suitable and use it to your benefit.

Exercise while on the Keto diet

Exercise is always recommended whether you are overweight or the right weight. You often hear people saying that you should add a little regular exercise to your everyday routine. Exercise will help you lose weight, get fit, stay healthy, look good, feel good, etc. All these are commonly associated benefits to exercise. When people want to lose weight, they usually start restricting the number of calories they consume and increase their exercise routine.

To see better results and more weight loss, increase your cardio and reduce calories in your diet. This overexertion leads to extreme fatigue, increased hunger, and mental exhaustion. This is why most diets fail to work for such people. This kind of approach is very generalized and not well researched. The stress put on the body makes you age faster, causes inflammation and is not sustainable.

Calories do count but not to the extent that you need to keep track of them with every bite you eat. When you follow the keto diet, you automatically reduce the carbs and protein and increase fat. This itself maintains a certain calorie balance that helps you lose weight due to ketosis. You might even know some people who have a fast metabolism such that even extra calories don't lead to weight gain in their body; however, this is not common so most people gain weight if they eat extra. The keto diet helps burn stored fat as carbs are burnt off fast. Low carb diets tend to give you a metabolic advantage. Another advantage over other diets is that it also helps to suppress your appetite. These aspects of the keto diet help you lose a lot of weight. You might think that adding exercise to this routine will help make it faster but you need to consider this carefully considering your health and lifestyle.

Sugar is one of the fastest sources of energy for our body and when we exercise, usually, it is the first fuel source that the body uses for energy; however, on a keto diet, access to this source is lost. This means that the body cannot function at the same high intensity as it was capable of before. After the glucose from carbs is burnt off, the body relies on glycolysis. Because of this, exercise that requires a lot of effort usually needs glucose as its energy source.

Ketones and fat cannot replace this glucose during exercise for the first few minutes. The pathways to burn fat and ketones only kick in after the first few minutes. The timing of the metabolic pathway will differ from person to person. Due to these factors, a ketogenic diet limits your performance in high-intensity exercise. Athletes who swim, undergo high-intensity interval training, play soccer, sprint, etc. cannot endure this on a ketogenic diet. These kinds of activities depend on glycolysis for energy. Heavy exercise also requires the correct amount of protein and fat to be consumed. If you are on a low carb diet, the other two macronutrients should be able to make up for it.

On a keto diet, highly active individuals need a good plan for macronutrient intake. Protein is given top priority here because fats and carbohydrates cannot make up for many of the protein's functions. Proteins stimulate muscle building, calorie burning and improve satiation, etc. Insufficient protein in your diet will also lead to loss of muscle mass and make you consume more calories. This will not help to lose weight and might even make you gain more.

Researchers recommend that there should be at least 2g of protein intake per kilogram of lean body mass for athletes and those who participate in heavy exercise. This helps to maintain or build muscle mass and burn fat. Higher protein intake is required on a keto diet because athletes use up excess protein to create glucose by gluconeogenesis. For such people, the best sources of keto proteins are eggs, meat, fish, low-carb protein powders and high-fat dairy.

In terms of carbs, you can determine it

according to your level of activity. You can start with 35g of carbs and try to lower it, if necessary. A targeted ketogenic diet is appropriate for individuals with such high-intensity activities so that they get the appropriate amount of all nutrients.

In terms of fat consumption while exercising, eat according to your goals. Those who want to lose weight should decrease fat calories to get a calorie deficit of around 500. Those who want to gain weight need to increase intake for a surplus of around 500 calories. You can always adjust the number according to your final goal.

For individuals who are affected by the carb deficit in a regular keto diet, the targeted or cyclic ketogenic diet is recommended. For those who are overweight and looking to lose weight, exercising on the normal keto diet will be beneficial. For those who practice regular endurance exercises, you can start with the usual keto recommendations. Watch the result for a week or two and adjust the diet a little to suit you better. If your endurance is not affected then keep your carbs to the recommended minimum of less than 35g per day. Exogenous ketones or MCTs can also be a good substitute for increasing carbs.

These tips are not the same for those who practice easier forms of exercise like regular jogging, aerobics, etc. A normal ketogenic diet works out fine for such activities unless you overdo it. There has to be a balance for everything you do. If you choose to add intermittent fasting to your keto diet lifestyle, I recommend avoiding exercise on days that you fast. Your energy levels are lower and might cause low blood pressure and dizziness if you exert yourself too much.

Otherwise, a little regular exercise is actually recommended. You can also take a break from exercise during the first few days of starting the keto diet. Let your body get adapted to a ketogenic diet slowly. Don't stress it out by making changes too fast and exerting it beyond its capability. After the initial adaptation, you can start exercising and might even notice an improvement in your endurance. For those who are obese and overweight, a better diet and regular exercise will definitely help you improve your stamina and endurance after a while.

Chapter Eight: Exercising on the Keto Diet For Overweight People Trying to Lose Weight

If you are not an athlete, the standard keto diet should be good enough for you. You can use exercise to improve your health and speed up the process of losing fat. This can be done with some simple regular cardio. You don't need to and shouldn't start practicing high-intensity sports that need sugar in your body. Just try a little jogging or running to increase your heart rate. The keto diet actually helps to improve performance in this kind of exercise. Your heart rate during the cardio session should be between 50% to 70% of your maximum heart rate. It can have many health benefits for you in the long run.

When you first start the keto diet, go for a slower pace. You can increase your speed or heart rate more in the next few weeks once your body is adapted to the keto diet. At this point, your body won't be dependent solely on carbs for energy during this type of exercise and will learn to utilize fat. For beginners who haven't exercised much before, try about 15 minutes of cardio in the first week. Increase this time by another 5 to 10 minutes every few days after that.

Soon you should be able to do at least 45 minutes of healthy cardio exercise every day. You can try cycling, running, circuit training, swimming, aerobics, etc. as your choice for this exercise. You might feel very tired when you first start out but your stamina and endurance will get much better if you keep at it. Cardio is a great way to speed up fat loss and improve the overall health of your body and especially your heart.

For Those Who Lift Weights

Just because you are on a diet does not mean that you cannot improve your strength or power and increase muscle mass. You can definitely do these in the keto diet. Your body doesn't require glucose for any activity that is less than 10 seconds long. Therefore, brief exertions on muscle by weightlifting will not be impaired by a ketogenic diet. As long as the sets are not longer than 10 seconds each, weightlifters can easily follow the keto diet and see an improvement in performance as well. The ideal program would have each exercise performed in five or less reps in five or lesser sets. This will help to increase strength as well as power within the ketogenic diet for weightlifters. Lower reps have been known to maximize muscle gain compared to higher reps; the appropriate volume is what is necessary.

Those who don't want to change their old programs can try carb supplements with their keto diet; however, carbs are not necessary to build muscle even though they prevent muscle breakdown. You can still gain muscle on a ketogenic diet as long as your protein and calorie intake is sufficient.

For Those Who Practice High-Intensity Sports Or Activities

The ketogenic diet can be beneficial for endurance athletes but not for those who play sports like soccer or basketball. It is useful for athletes who are trying to lose weight and get in shape, but performance-wise, at least in the initial stage, it will decrease the ability of the performer. People who play sports like golf can easily follow the ketogenic diet, but for sports like rugby and soccer, the body is dependent on the glycolytic pathway for energy. The keto diet will harm the performance of such sportspersons. Easily digestible carbohydrates are a better source of energy for these kinds of sports.

In case of boxing or wrestling, keto dieting helps to lose water weight. Athletes can also choose to follow the keto diet during off seasons when they don't have to perform and need to watch their weight more carefully. Hence, any sport that requires short bursts of energy is suited for a keto diet.

There are many supplements that athletes, sportsmen and anyone who exercises can use during a ketogenic diet:

• Beta-alanine is a supplement suitable for bodybuilders or high-intensity athletes who rely on the glycolytic pathway.

- Taurine is a supplement that has shown to improve exercise performance and decrease fatigue.

- Caffeine supplements help due to its stimulatory effect and increased cortisol levels.

- Exogenous ketones are a source of instant energy and recommended for endurance athletes or cardio training.

- MCT's or Medium Chain Triglycerides are saturated fat supplements, which are also good for endurance athletes and cardio trainers.

- Creatine is the perfect supplement for anyone who wants to increase muscle mass and strength and is ideal for weightlifters.

- Protein powders like casein, whey, collagen, etc. help to get the required protein intake according to an individual's needs.

- Alpha GPC is said to enhance growth hormone secretion, power output, etc and is ideal for weightlifters and athletes.

- Fish oil is a commonly recommended supplement, which helps to stimulate muscle protein synthesis and boosts the process of recovery. L-Citrulline is ideal for most athletes other than golfers or powerlifters because it reduces fatigue and improves endurance.

Depending on the purpose of the supplement, you can get any that you particularly need for your body.

Chapter Nine: Following the Keto Diet While Traveling or Eating Out

Now let's talk about what to do when you are traveling or just out with your friends. You can go and have fun without compromising on your keto diet. There are days where you can cheat and not be too strict with yourself; however, if you tend to go out a lot, it is important to learn how to stay keto-friendly on those days as well.

Keeping your meal low on carbohydrates is not difficult at all. There are some easy tips that will help you stick with the diet no matter where you go:

• The first thing to remember is to pass on starchy foods like bread, pasta, and potatoes. It might be tempting but this will undo all your efforts to lose weight. Order a meal without starchy foods that are not keto-friendly. For this, we recommend ordering something like a salad as an appetizer. If you like eating burgers for lunch, substitute the buns for lettuce leaves or any green leaf that appeals to you. Most restaurants will accommodate this request quite willingly and if they don't, just give your buns to your friend to enjoy. Also, try to avoid pizza if you can't resist the crust. The toppings of any pizza are usually keto friendly but not the crust. If you order a plate of something that still has starchy sides, pass it on to your friend or just don't touch it if you have enough self-control. Making some simple requests at a restaurant can be done easily and they will cooperate better if you suggest medical issues.

• Don't ignore the sauces and condiments with your meal. Some sauces can actually be loaded with the carbs that you are trying to avoid. Read up on the ingredients or simply ask for them. Stick to fatty sauces like béarnaise and stay away from the ketchup bottle.

• Add fat to your meal if there isn't enough. This can easily be done by asking for some butter, olive oil or other keto friendly ingredients. You can even carry some small packs of these yourself when you go out. Adding this extra fat will make you feel much more satisfied with the meal you eat.

• Try to avoid desserts as much as you can. Most of the time, this last part of the meal contains way too much sugar and is bad for your diet. If you must have dessert, opt for something like berries with some heavy cream or a cheese plate. If you can avoid it, just drink some tea or coffee while the others have their dessert.

• Learn to improvise. Getting creative is the best option for you if the place you go to is not keto friendly. Talk to the waiter or chef and improvise on the items on the menu. Instead of the spaghetti, just ask for the sauce with some vegetables and cheese on top. This can be your very own dish for dinner.

Or you could just order a few keto friendly appetizers and avoid carb loaded main dishes. Work with what they have and as long as your requests aren't too fussy, most places will willingly accommodate their customers.

• Don't give in to temptation even if you are at a huge buffet with everything that you like eating. Stay away from dishes that have potatoes and grains in particular. Also, avoid the dessert table. As long as you follow these basics, there will still be a lot of dishes that you can load on your plate. Eat more salads, seafood, vegetables, and meat. Choose dressings like sour cream and olive oil for healthy fats. If you are trying to lose weight, don't get carried away at buffets and start with a small plate of food. If you really feel hungry after you are done, just go back for seconds. There is no need to pile a mountain of food out of greed that you will later feel guilty about.

• If your friends or family have invited you over for dinner, try to let them know in advance about what you can and cannot eat. Help them out by suggesting some easy substitutes for your meal and, in this way, they will not be inconvenienced at the last moment. No one likes a guest who comes over and fusses about the food. If you really cannot do this, just make an excuse like a stomachache instead of talking about your diet.

- Another way to avoid overeating at restaurants is by eating a little keto snack at home before you go out. This will take the edge off for you so that you don't indulge in carb foods at the restaurant trying to fill your stomach up.

- If you are going to a fast food joint, just try to cut out some items - this will make all the difference. For instance, skip the soda or fries. Load up on toppings for your burger or sandwich and choose your dressing carefully. You can have some mayo or normal mustard sauce. Don't order ketchup or flavored mustard sauces or barbeque sauce. Don't order fried chicken and opt for grilled meat instead. Ditch the bread and use leaves or salads with your meal.

- While choosing a place to eat out, you can just pick the most keto-friendly places to go to in advance. Mexican food will work if you avoid the tortilla chips. Burrito bowls are a great option with no rice and are loaded with meat and vegetables. Add guacamole and a ton of cheese and sour cream and it's a perfect keto bowl. If they don't provide burrito bowls, just take off the wrap and eat the filling. Asian restaurants can be a bit of a problem since rice and noodles are a staple for these cuisines. Order dishes that are made with brown sauce, coconut oil, sesame oil or any such good fat. Stay away from sweet sauces and thickeners. Eat stir-fries with more meat and veggies. Indian food can actually be quite keto friendly. There are many meat dishes cooked in creamy sauces, dishes with vegetables other than potato, kebabs, etc.

All the above tips will help you in deciding what to eat when you are away from home. There is no reason to exclude yourself from fun gatherings as long as you learn how to control your food habits. Avoiding carbs in dishes is very simple. There's no need to panic while you're at restaurants or traveling anymore. Any place in the world can provide you with a keto-friendly meal if you know how to pick right.

Conclusion

For years, you might have been taught how certain ways to eat are right or wrong and told that all kinds of fat are bad for you. The word fat itself has been given a very negative title that makes it seem like the one causing weight issues. All the weight loss diets you have tried over the years have probably asked you to cut out all fats and count your calories every time you eat something, but now, you know better. This book was created to help you understand how there are good kinds of fat that are beneficial for your body and will help you lose weight.

Once you understand how ketosis works, you know that the recipes and ingredients in a keto diet will help you get in shape and not gain weight. The keto diet might seem radically different to you right now but a hundred years ago it was the norm for your ancestors. And they were definitely leading a much healthier lifestyle than we are.

Our modern diet is bent toward a very unhealthy processed diet that can lead to many health issues. Those who believe the stigma of fat will still be counting calories and not seeing any change in their weight. Changing your mindset is the first thing that will help you learn more about your body and get it back to a healthy state.

I hope this book has helped you understand the role of fat in your body and how the keto diet will help you much more than any other fad diet.

You need to remember that sugar and processed food is very unhealthy and not something your ancestors would ever eat. Even while we advance in other fields, you need to remember that our bodies would still prefer the basic diet that it was accustomed to before. Use the tips given in this book and you can easily start a healthy keto lifestyle. It is simple to maintain this diet for a long time and feasible even when you go out for meals or are traveling.

Within a few weeks of trying the keto diet, you will see how your body burns up excess fat and gets in shape. You will feel more alert and have the energy to go about your daily tasks better. A good diet can have a huge positive impact on your life. If you found this book useful, I ask that you to recommend it to friends or family who could use the extra help too.

References

https://www.healthline.com/nutrition/ketogenic-diet-101
https://charliefoundation.org/diet-plans/
https://factvsfitness.com/paleo-vs-atkins-vs-ketogenic-diet/
https://perfectketo.com/simple-tips-for-staying-keto-while-youre-on-vacation/
https://www.ruled.me/complete-guide-exercise-ketogenic-diet/